W9-DJI-193

Lincoln School Library

The Let's Talk Library™

Let's Talk About Smoking

Elizabeth Weitzman

The Rosen Publishing Group's
PowerKids Press™
New York

For Sydelle Gugick Weitzman

Published in 1996 by The Rosen Publishing Group, Inc.
29 East 21st Street, New York, NY 10010

First Edition

Book design: Erin McKenna

Photo credits: Cover, pp. 4, 8, 11, 12, 15 by Maria Moreno; p. 16 by Sarah Friedman; p. 19 © Steve Easton/International Stock; p. 20 © Dusty Willison/International Stock.

Weitzman, Elizabeth.
 Let's talk about smoking / Elizabeth Weitzman. — 1st ed.
   p. cm. — (The let's talk library)
 Includes index.
 Summary: Discusses the dangers of smoking and ways to avoid starting this habit.
 ISBN 0-8239-2307-X
 1. Stepfamilies—Juvenile literature. [1. Stepfamilies.] I. Title. II. Series.
 HV5733.W35 1996
 362.29'6—dc20   96-14327
                          CIP
                          AC

Manufactured in the United States of America

Table of Contents

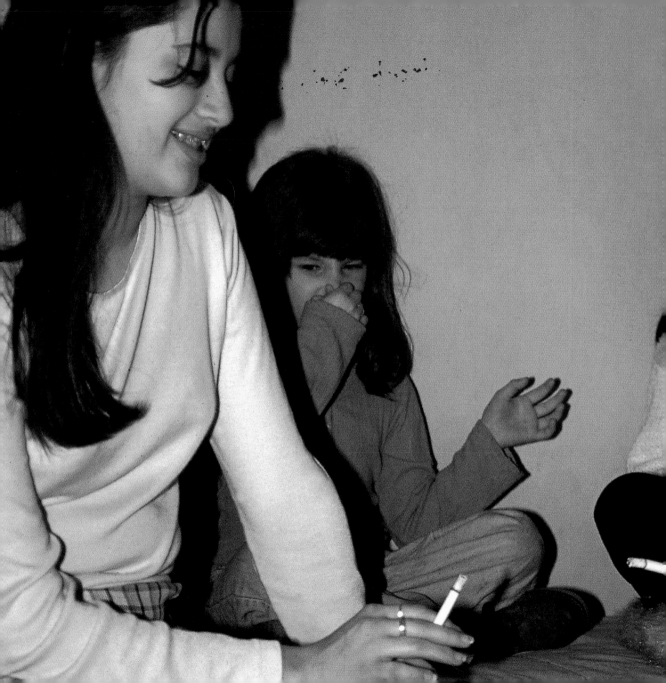

Janie

Janie coughed and opened the window in her big sister Deena's room. "Why do you have to smoke?" she asked Deena.

"All my friends do," Deena answered. "Besides, it looks cool."

Janie shook her head. "I think it's pretty stupid."

"What do you know?" Deena said as Janie walked out the door. Actually, Janie knew a lot more than Deena.

◀ Many teens smoke because their friends do.

Where Do Cigarettes Come From?

Cigarettes (sih-gar-ETZ) and **cigars** (sih-GARZ) are made from a plant called **tobacco** (tuh-BACK-oh). Like corn and tomatoes, tobacco plants are grown on farms. The plants are picked and sent to factories that turn them into cigarettes or cigars. Then the cigarettes or cigars are packaged and sent to stores for people to buy. But unlike corn and tomatoes, tobacco hurts your body. In fact, cigarettes are so bad for you that every pack has a warning label on it.

There is a warning label on every pack of cigarettes. ▶

8 mg "tar." 0.7 mg nicotine av per cigarette by FTC method

SURGEON GENERAL'S WARNING: Smoking Causes Lung Cancer, Heart Disease, Emphysema, And May Complicate Pregnancy.

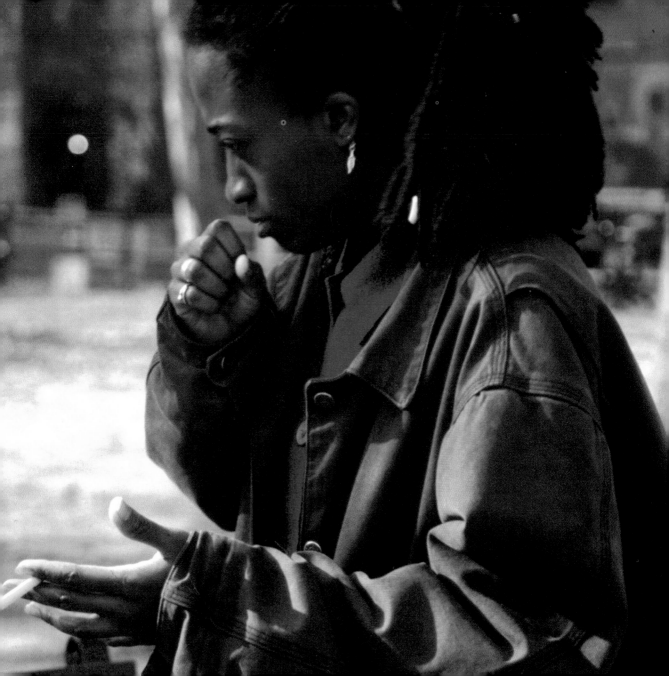

What's So Bad About Smoking?

When a person smokes, she breathes in tar. The tar stays in her body and sticks to her lungs. This makes it harder for her to breathe. After many years, the tar will cover most of her lungs. Cigarettes also contain hundreds of poisons. Many of these poisons cause cancer, a disease that makes people very sick and can even be **fatal** (FAY-tul).

When a person stops smoking, her body tries to heal itself. Some of the damage can be fixed, and some can't.

◀ A person who smokes may cough a lot to try to clear her lungs of tar.

Secondhand Smoke

Cigarettes are bad for everyone, not just people who smoke. First, someone decides to light a cigarette. Then he passes on the bad stuff to you by blowing his smoke into the air you breathe. This is called **second-hand** (SEK-end-hand) smoke.

Secondhand smoke is very harmful. In many places people are not allowed to smoke at all. This way, you won't be hurt by all the poisons from other people's cigarettes.

Breathing in someone else's smoke is almost as bad for you as smoking is. ▶

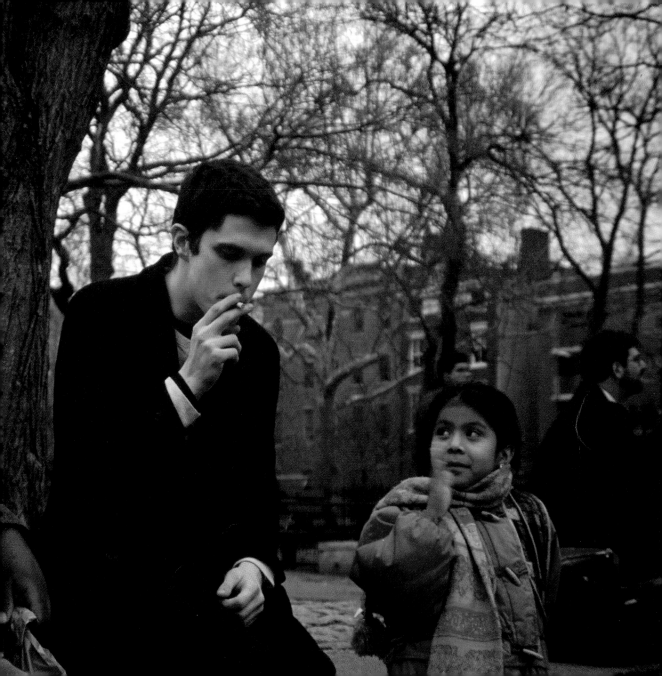

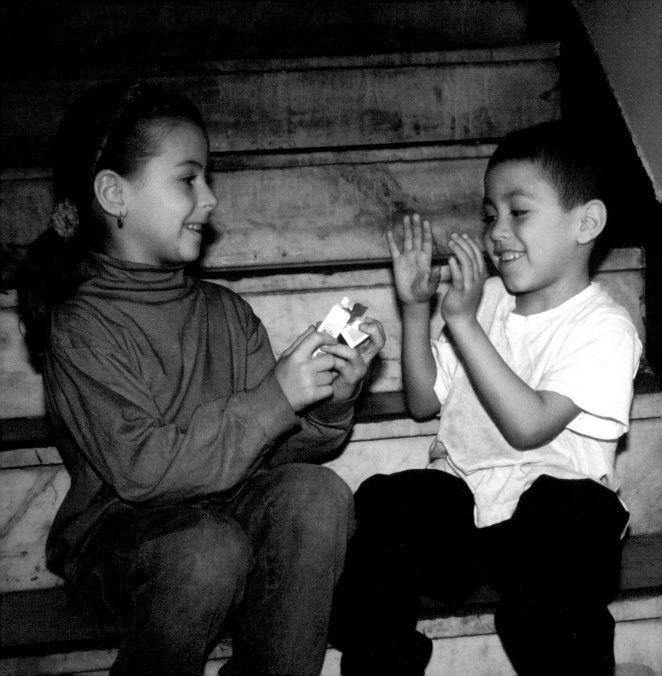

Why Do Kids Smoke?

Most kids start smoking because other kids push them to. It's not always easy to say no, especially to your friends. But if you say yes to smoking, you also say yes to all the dangers of cigarettes.

The best way to handle **pressure** (PREH-sher) from friends is to say, "No, thanks," as calmly as you can, even if you're nervous. After all, you really *don't* want all the bad things that come with smoking.

◄ You can practice saying no to cigarettes with a friend.

13

Cigarette Ads

Cigarette ads can also **influence** (IN-flu-ents) kids to smoke. They usually show beautiful people doing fun things, or tough cowboy types, or cartoon characters like Joe Camel. But cigarettes don't make you beautiful or tough or help you have fun. They give you bad breath, yellow teeth, and wrinkles. And they can make you very sick. Not only that, but it's illegal to buy them unless you're an adult. Once you know the facts, you'll be too smart to be fooled by these ads.

Using cartoon characters, such as Joe Camel, is one way cigarette makers get kids' attention. ▶

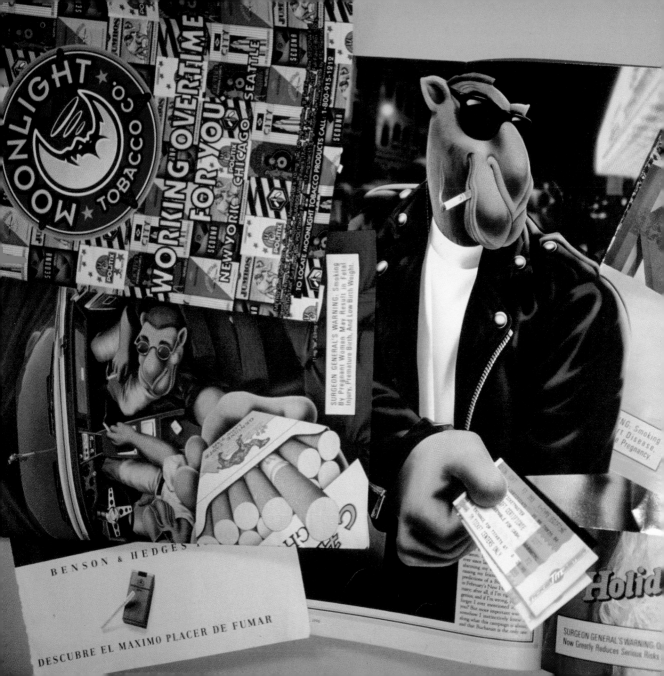

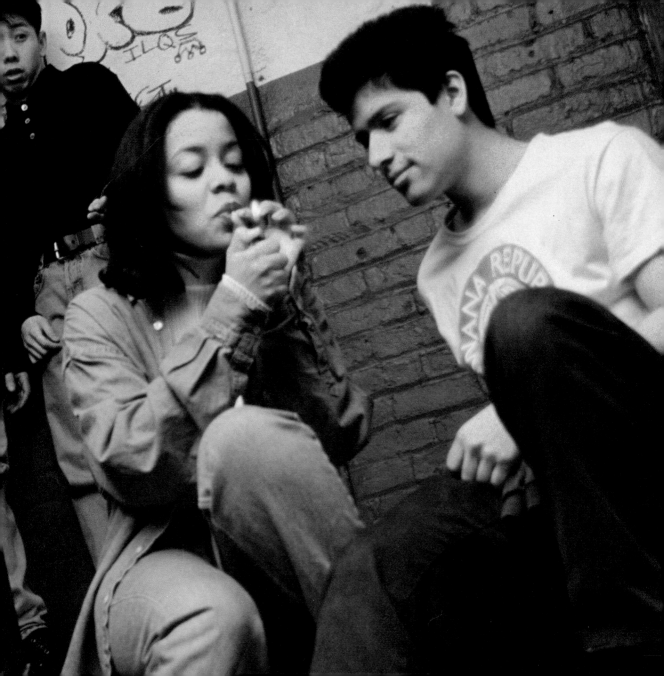

Why Do Grown-ups Smoke?

Most adults know that cigarettes are dangerous. So why do many of them smoke? Because a chemical called **nicotine** (NIK-o-teen) is in every cigarette. Nicotine is very **addictive** (a-DIK-tiv). This means that once your body gets used to it, it **craves** (KRAYVZ), or needs, it.

Nicotine makes a person's heart beat too fast. In the beginning, this might just make her feel nervous. After many years of smoking, though, it can damage her heart.

◄ **Many teens start smoking before they realize how hard it is to stop.**

17

If Your Parents Smoke

If your parents smoke, there is a greater chance that you will too. It makes sense that if you love and respect people, you will want to be like them. But your parents probably started smoking before people knew how unsafe cigarettes were. Now that you know, you can choose not to smoke. And one day your parents might even decide to stop smoking.

A parent who chooses not to smoke sets a healthy example for his child. ▶

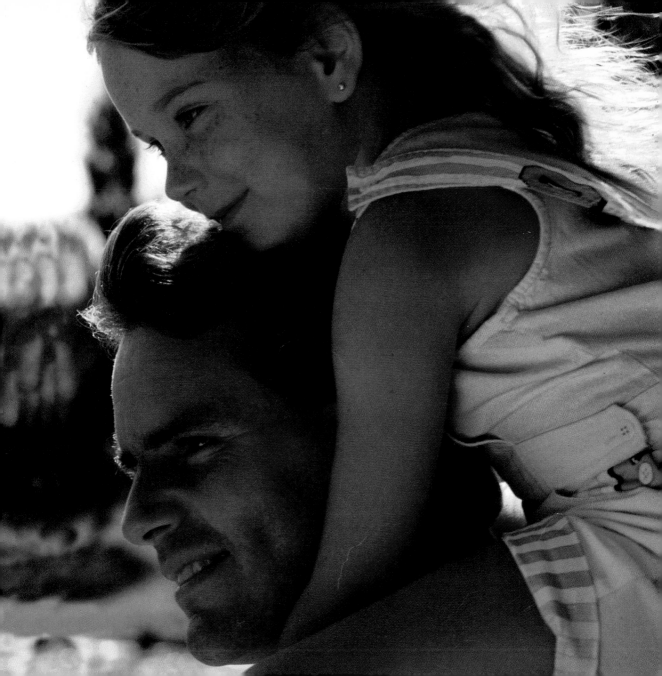

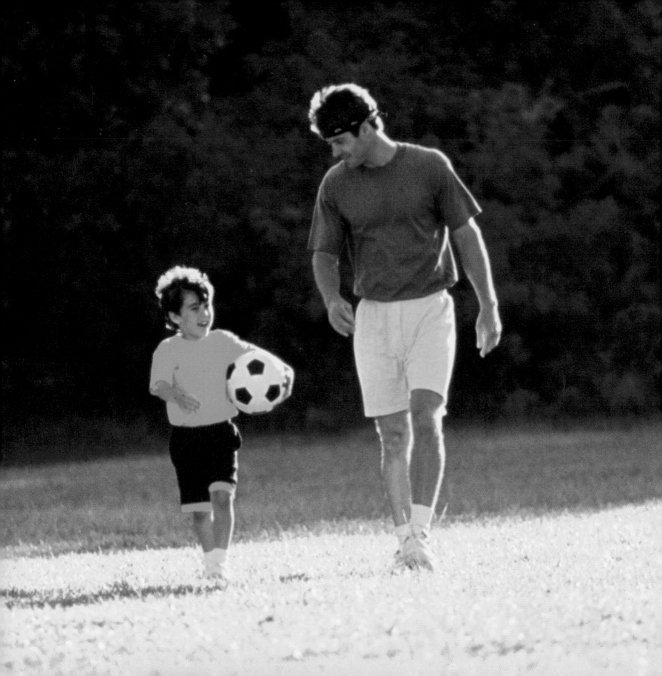

Quitting Smoking

Since nicotine is addictive, it is not easy to give up cigarettes.

But there are lots of ways to help someone stop smoking. If your parent wants to quit, find something you can do together. Do you collect baseball cards? Get your dad interested. He might even have some old ones hidden away. Sharing a hobby may help keep his mind off of smoking. And you'll get to spend some extra time with him.

◀ Sharing a hobby or a sport with your dad
may help take his mind off of smoking.

Nothing Cool About It

Smoking poisons the air and everyone who breathes that air. It hurts a person's lungs, it is bad for his heart, and it can cause cancer.

Cigarettes cost a lot of money. They're addictive, so the smoker has a hard time giving them up. They stain fingers and teeth, and they make people smell bad.

Would you really call that cool?

Glossary

addictive (a-DIK-tiv) Creating a strong craving.

cigar (sih-GAR) Coarsely shredded tobacco rolled in heavy, dark paper.

cigarette (sih-gar-ET) Finely shredded tobacco rolled in thin paper.

crave (KRAYV) Needing something.

fatal (FAY-tul) Causing death.

influence (IN-flu-ents) Having an affect on how someone acts.

nicotine (NIK-o-teen) Chemical in tobacco.

pressure (PREH-sher) To make a person feel as though he or she must do something.

secondhand (SEK-end-hand) Belonging to someone else first.

tobacco (tuh-BACK-oh) Plant that is usually smoked.

23

Index

362.29   Weitzman, Elizabeth.
WEI
        Let's talk about
        smoking